# Driven by Depression

### True stories of people finding light in the darkness

### plus opinions of Health Care & other professionals

by

## Hana Rubinstejnova

*This book is dedicated to all those who ever experienced some form of depression and learned to overcome the symptoms. It is also dedicated to those who ever encountered someone who suffered with depression. Your life became richer for that experience. And of course to those who suffered and could not get out of depression without taking their own life. May their soul find peace.*

ISBN 978-1-326-50178-5

## TABLE OF CONTENTS

Acknowledgement

Endorsement

Author's Note

CHAPTER 1

Author's Experiences with Depression

- My History
- First Onset of Depression
- Second Onset of Depression
- Third Onset of Depression
- How did I get motivated and inspired about life again?
- What Worked for Me and My Personal Recommendations

CHAPTER 2

Other people's personal stories

- Lynn
- Alohana
- Tracy
- Renee
- E.G.
- J.L.
- Carol
- Andrea
- Aldwyn
- Robin
- Dr. Alejandro
- Linda
- Chris
- Danna
- Jeannette

## CHAPTER 3

Health Care Professionals on Depression

- Dr Thomas Stone
- Mike Carey
- Mary McKennan LMT
- Kathy Cash RN, CHPD
- Jeffrey Briar
- Arnold Wiseman
- Sherwood Grant
- Chuck Bluestein
- Karen Polvinale
- Thomas Hiatt, CWC, CPT, CNC, PT
- Carol Leek
- Patricia L McGuire MD

## CHAPTER 4

Good Resources

- About Depression
- Overcoming Depression

ABOUT THE AUTHOR

## ENDORSEMENT

"Hana's book is filled with useful facts and ideas for those struggling with depression. Hana's writing is clear and this book is easy to follow. It includes lots of professional perspectives will be helpful to anyone dealing with depression (or their loved ones.) Thomas Hiatt's practical suggestions prove true in my experience as well. I recommend this book."

*Tim Hallbom MSW*
*President, NLP and Coaching institute, Inc.*

## AUTHOR'S NOTE

It is important to understand that depression doesn't choose only the less fortunate of people. There are too many in the history of mankind who suffered with depression and who were accomplished celebrities with all one can ask for in a matter of material possessions. What money cannot buy is the internal experience and peaceful mind.

Some of these famous celebrities are Alan Alda, Woody Allen, Julian Assange, Alec Baldwin, Ingmar Bergman, Jon Bon Jovi, Barbara Bush, Jim Carrey, Ray Charles, Agatha Christie, Windston Churchill, Eric Clapton, Leonard Cohen, Charles Darwin, Johnny Depp, Diana Princess of Wales, Charles Dickens, Bob Dylan, Eminem, Harrison Ford, Paul Gauguin, Paul Getty, Audrey Hepburn, Sir Anthony Hopkins, Janet Jackson, Angelina Jolie, Franz Kafka, Alicia Keys, Stephen King, Kurt Cobain, John Lennon, Ewan McGregor, Michelangelo, Marilyn Monroe, Isaac Newton, Gwyneth Paltrow, Brad Pitt, Edgar Allan Poe, Bruce Springsteen, Uma Thurman, Leo Tolstoy, Mark Twain, Vincent van Gogh, Walt Whitman, Robbie Williams, Robin Williams, Oprah Winfrey and many other professionals – see: http://en.wikipedia.org/wiki/List_of_people_with_major_depressive_disorder

This book consists of personal events from my own life, life stories from other people who suffered with depression and various points of view of many health professionals. My purpose for this book is to portray a true picture about the effects of depression and some common misconceptions about it in public eye.

May this book bring more light into many lives.

The Author

CHAPTER 1

## MY PERSONAL EXPERIENCE

### My history

There was nothing in my upbringing that would suggest that I would suffer from depression in my life. There is no history of mental illness in our family, neither any history of depression in the extended family. Yet, as you might agree, that still doesn't mean anything.

Depression is not picky. It can affect anyone. The onset of depression can be triggered by sudden change of circumstances that the individual is unable to handle with ease.

My first experience with depression occured in late 2008 when my professional life circumstances changed. Until then I was a rather successful professional working for a corporation that provided both work challenges as well as safety of a stable position.

However, during the last few years before that I engaged in a massive dose of personal development. I went through a variety of trainings in the natural health fields and other professional and business related trainings. I used to attend every possible seminar I could get my hands on.

Whether it was related to coaching, healing, online marketing, promotion and business strategies, I attended all of them. At every one of them I filled the various workbooks with copious notes and was fully charged up and ready to roll. That was the idea anyway. Before the end of 2008 I decided to leave the safety net of the corporate world and start up my own healing therapy venture.

With all sorts of qualifications behind my belt, I thought that was all that was necessary for a success in business. And then the time came when I was at home every day, putting hours of work into the marketing and other business aspects of my new role as a healer and coach.

## First Onset of Depression

After seeing some clients, I realized I wasn't ready. I had a massive amount of self-doubt and fears and I was unable to move forward in my business. And that was the time when depression 'hit' me for the first time.

That time it came in a rather 'light' form. I was not motivated enough to do anything and I slept a lot. This bout of depression took a few months. Then I started to read books again. I immersed myself into some spiritual books, looking for the meaning of life and what to do next. I slowly became functioning again.

During the year 2009 I was looking for ways to grow and to improve as a human being and a quality professional. Once I 'accidentally' came across a Vipassana meditation retreat and met a few people who have had done it. I felt drawn towards it myself. It sounded great and challenging enough and I wanted to experience the bliss of deep meditation and profound insights.

It seemed to be good enough so I decided to sign up for it. The rules and restrictions imposed on participants of the retreat didn't deter me from giving it a go. It was held towards the end of the year in one of the Vipassana international centers in Australia.

It went to be a truly life changing experience for me without a doubt. It was an experience that I would not wish to anyone. Despite the fact that for eight out of the ten days at the retreat I felt amazing and ecstatic. At the end it turned out to be rather dramatic experience that led to many other dramatic events in the following years.

After the retreat I had an urge to write about my experience at the retreat and it created a very personal and detailed book that still has not been traditionally published for a fear of being publicly ridiculed. I will not go into much more details here. Enough is to say that I ended up in hospital's high dependency unit for a few days.

This dramatic experience led to a number of others during the following year. The reason I am describing all the above is to paint a picture about what events in my life were the catalyst for the depression.

## Second Onset of Depression

My second experience with depression took place in the second half of 2010 when I was again hospitalized and had to take a medication that I know had a direct suppressing effect on my feelings and motivation. While I was still in hospital I fell into a deep depression. Everything lost its meaning and purpose. Life was a drag. Only with strong willpower I was able to overcome the side effects of this drug to the point that I eventually presented well enough to be let go home.

The symptoms of depression persisted for long time that time. I was withdrawn, wasn't motivated or inspired to do anything, lacked appetite, moved in a slow motion, and had experienced a variety of other signs.

It was a rather challenging time for me and my family. Although I did have a loving support from both, my partner and my parents, nobody seemed to understand my perspective. I felt very alone amongst love and care.

During the next few months my condition was rather stagnant and so under the doctor's pressure I reluctantly agreed to try antidepressants. I was very careful and observant about any changes that would be occuring to me after being on these pills.

I was taking them for one month and as I did not feel better at all and was more worried about the side and long term effects of these drugs, I resisted the doctor's recommendation to give them more time and stopped taking them.

Around that time I agreed to try natural methods of combating depression and did a Narrative Therapy and Counselling. They both have helped a bit in some respect. If not in overcoming the depression symptoms, then at least in distracting me and providing me with something to be engaged in.
Looking at it now in a long term perspective this also gave me the opportunity to see how these professions operate.

I slowly but surely regained some of my strengths back with more time. The depression started to lose hold of me in 2011. The following 2 years were great. I had some motivation again, I felt successful, contributed and had a purpose.

## Third Onset of Depression

Then in 2013 I got another opportunity for a growth from the Universe. This time it was the worst experience of my life. I suddenly lost control of my mind and body and as the events got worse, I received a very harsh medical treatment. I was devastated on all levels: the body, mind and soul. I felt crushed completely.

These events led to my third and worst case of depression in my life. This time it was really serious. I lost all life meaning and was very tired during the day. The only thing I 'loved' was sleeping and dreaming. In my dreams life was good and I was invincible. In reality I suffered in silence.

At awakening each morning my mind was devastated to find out I was still alive and had to tackle another day on this planet. It was extremely soul wrenching exercise to go through that every day.

There was nothing missing in my life. I had all I needed to feel great; all the resources were freely available to me. I should have felt loved and appreciated and wealthy and supported and all that. Yet, I didn't care. It was almost meaningless. I lost touch with life's benefits. I wished to be dead.

It was a deep soul searching exercise for me. It took me many months to get out of it. I tried Psychology & Cognitive Behavior Therapy that time, yet after many months I still couldn't see any significant success with it.

I was opposed to taking antidepressants again as I don't like to take drugs. Especially those that have significant side effects, which can be even worse than the condition that they try to treat.

## How did I get motivated and inspired about life again?

Some things that I did to recover from depression follow. Once I was able to do it, I immersed my mind in uplifting, positive messages from the Internet. I researched online for inspiring quotes, motivating videos and uplifting presentations. I followed people who inspired me. I networked with loving and compassionate individuals and I surrounded myself with supportive friends and family.

I walked a lot. I got together with my amazing neighbour a few times a week and we walked the neighborhood for hours. It was a very important part of my recovery process. Not only did I spend time outside and moved my body. I also learned a great deal about another person's life story. It has been a very supportive friendship.

Another thing that helped me to escape the depressive moods is the fact that I traveled overseas to see my country of origin. It was a very reconnecting experience. One that helped me to get a new perspective on my life and on myself. On my return to Australia I felt much better. Although I felt disconnected with Australia after spending some time with my family and friends, I decided to take action again.

As previously in my life I was drawn towards helping others with my skills and life experiences. Not only that other people are helped, but I also feel fulfillment in the process of helping them. I started to connect the dots and soon it all came together. I realized how much I do love to coach and help people to transform. After more encouraging comments from my peers and friends I took action and started with coaching again.

Since the moment I realized that I know what I love to do in this life I got more energy, clearer mind, more focus, determination and inspiration to be the best I can be. Although it was motivated from without, the source of this action was the inspiration from within.

The fact that I'm now putting together this book speaks volumes about my rediscovered abilities, especially the ability to focus and get things done.

## What Worked for Me and My Personal Recommendations

There surely were various factors in both, my environment and my personality, that aided in the recovery process. The fact that I was loved by my family and friends enough to let me find a way to live my passion and a fulfilling life helped enormously. When I was getting out of the worst of depression's symptoms, I realized just how much my condition depended on the support of others.

The life long lasting relationships that I sustain with my family members and friends were of the most benefit to me. It was important for me to be able to share my concerns, worries and fears with others who loved me despite the debilitating condition I suffered with.

They might not had been through the same life experience and might not have fully understood the way I felt and thought, however, they were there for me when I needed them most.

To give you an example, I would be seeing my parents (who live in Europe) via Skype almost on a daily basis. Although there wasn't much I would say during the video call, I would listen to them talking to me. Even when I wasn't able to concentrate fully on the full conversation, I still persisted and stayed connected.

Just the feeling of connection with another human being, especially one who loves you unconditionally was very important for me. It made me feel a little more connected and not alone. And also it helped me when I was having suicidal thoughts. The main reason I didn't act upon the long term thoughts was that I felt responsible and loved.

One thing that I was telling myself to help me deal with the thoughts of suicide was this: "I can always commit a suicide. There is no rush, but at least wait for the time when I don't have anyone who loves me and who would be devastated by it. Perhaps do it when life is really hard on me and I have absolutely nothing. Now is not that time. Let's wait." That was my rather twisted thought process.

I am kind of proud of myself now. I am proud of my determination and perhaps even a bit of courage to not rely on medication to get better, but to be able to overcome depression on my own terms, rather than succumbing to the so common dose of doctors' advice. Maybe there is a certain place for medication to alleviate the symptoms of depression, but I was too concerned about the probable side effects, especially long term ones, with use of these prescription drugs.

To be able to win the 'fight' (even though I don't like this aggressive word too much) with depression it is important to look at all the aspects of ones' life. Whether it's physical activity, food and drinks consumption, environmental factors, mental activity and thought processing, social interaction, family support and other lifestyle factors, they all form the basis of being well and thriving.

However, finding one's purpose and passion in life is the most uplifting and natural healing method for depression. At least in my opinion.

Nevertheless, I don't discount the fact that diet and exercise have a place in overcoming depression. However, I have been on mostly natural plant based lifestyle for over 7 years and yet I suffered with depression anyway. Still I would recommend a well balanced natural diet to people who suffer with depression as that may help to harmonize their body energies and can help to overcome the side effects of potential medication.

Depression is best tackled with support. If you find yourself being depressed for prolonged periods of time, please seek help. It can be as simple as asking your family and friends for a chat. Share your thoughts, feelings, and emotions with people who will listen to your story.

If there is nobody in your family and friend's circles, find a professional. They are there for the very purpose to help you find the way back to living a purposeful life. There are services that can be accessed for free (some by referral) and there are other paid ones. Whatever you can afford, there is an option.

Check some resources at the end of this book for some ideas. Be well.

## CHAPTER 2

## OTHER PEOPLE'S STORIES ABOUT DEPRESSION

### LYNN'S STORY

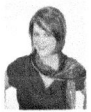

Lynn Hope Thomas M.Sc.
Author and Change Lead, Demartini Facilitator
www.breakingthroughloss.com

Depression for me was an ever increasing sense of despair as I experienced one tragic event after another. Not that each event was more tragic than the loss of my sisters but it felt like an escalating build up, with an underlying confusion over the decades. Every time I stood up and recovered I was knocked down again.

**Back in 1972**

I was nine years old when I experienced the loss of my sisters. I call it my personal 9/11 as they were 11 years old. They died within a month of each other, and back in 1972 no-one talked to children about how they felt about loss, let alone losing two siblings.

As a result my grief was kept internal, I stifled the emotion and because the emotion was 'trapped' in my body, it actually set me up to reproduce scenarios in my life that would aim at drawing the emotion out. These events began to depress me.

**Roll Forward 2010**

In the year 2010, I was losing my energy, I was a single parent with a young daughter to care for. I worked full-time; having left the United Kingdom to start a 'new life' in Australia following a traumatic divorce; I was now under the threat of redundancy.

I was so tired of my bad luck in life and tired of living. I would never take an 'exit' strategy though I would think about it. You see life was simply no fun at all. I could not see what enjoyment could come.......based on my past experiences it was just filled with struggle, grief and a distinct lack of pleasure. I had a little dog and I just did not have the energy to get up earlier in a morning and take her for a walk before heading off to work. I felt quite pathetic, and because I felt pathetic I simply couldn't share that thought with anyone. I don't know why, I simply couldn't talk about my feelings to anyone I knew.

## Traditional Support

I went to the Doctor's knowing she would tell me I was depressed and yes she would prescribe me some pills. How could pills make me feel different about my life? You know ...how could they give me more energy? The Doctor assigned me to talk to a psychologist.

I can't honestly say to myself I was depressed, but then if someone told me that they felt that they didn't want to live, saw no joy in life and didn't want to get out of bed, then even I would have to say they were depressed. The job of the psychologist was to listen and guide me, but when she heard of the traumatic events in my life then even she had to agree that one would emotionally be challenged.

Just as I started talking with the psychologist, I attended a course in Brisbane called the Breakthrough Experience. A friend had recommended me going to it, and I said yes! On reflection, it seems a little crazy because firstly she knew nothing about my condition and little about my life and secondly it was a relatively expensive course.

I went willingly, trusting the recommendation and with the sentiment that I knew, very much so, that I wanted to change how I saw things in my life. I was ready for change.

## Life Changing Breakthrough

That weekend in Brisbane changed my life forever. I came back home and felt for the first time in a long time truly inspired. Inspired to take action on what I had learnt and I wanted to find a way to share it.

Over the next few weeks my brain was tingling, I felt as if there were fireworks lighting up in my brain, so much so it would awaken me at night. When I had my next appointment with the psychologist, she sat and listened intently as I explained to her I was not depressed, my energy was back! Smiling and full of energy I told her that I didn't need to talk with her anymore, that there were others who needed her help now. Yes! I was going to write a book about it and share the discovery with others.

I could see she had 'caring' suspicions. You can imagine can't you, what might have been going through her mind? Yes! She might think I was mad. She was lovely; she asked me to call her if I felt differently at any point but told me she was pleased for me.

Following that day, my life did not suddenly become easier or less 'taskful', but what had changed significantly was my attitude and also the feeling of inspiration by deciding to embark on something which I highly valued. I began writing my book called 'Breaking Through Loss'.

Thanking you for reading up to this point, I really don't want to be talking about myself so much, because if you are reading this book, clearly you have been attracted to it because you want to learn more about depression and how to transcend it.

I commend truly Hana for being inspired to write this book and pull together views and opinions from different people, all for the benefit of others. There is never only one way to a solution, you just need to find the one that resonates with you the most. Everyone has a different reason for their depression.

**Alternative recovery**

I can now share some of what I have learnt about Depression. The main lessons have been learnt by training as a Facilitator of the Demartini Method, after reaching a profound insight into the cycles of repeat over the decades. Please note that I do not advocate anyone to ignore their own Doctor's medical advice.

Depression arises when we have unrealistic expectations about an event, a situation, or another person's actions. Depression results from an addiction to one or more fantasies or delusions about how things are supposed to be. Note here to listen to any 'Should Be' & 'Should Haves' as this indicates a fantasy and how one may be ignoring the facts of how things actually are.

When reality does not match the fantasy we will feel sad or depressed. When more positives are stacked up against the negatives in our mind, the fantasy will create the polar opposite, and we experience the emotions of depression. It is the desire of the unattainable which feeds our suffering and the degree to which this happens depends upon the strength of the fantasy/delusion in terms of the ratio of positives to negatives.

As a trained Demartini Facilitator, through the use of the Breakthrough technique the depressed individual can be guided to balance out the ratio's and once that is done the depression dissolves. have witnessed many people alleviate loss and grief, depression, victimization, as well as helped many too, including myself.

My book is a testimony to the science of the method. My life now is very different, that is not to say that I can now avoid or never experience a depression, or suffer from grief of a loss.

What it does mean is that I now have a tool I can use which will allow me to see the beauty of the situation, and relieve myself of those often painful and negative emotions. And if I don't work through it myself I know I can find a Demartini Facilitator to help. That is my choice, and one I will always take from now on.

In my story I show clearly the events and cycles that my imbalanced perceptions created, these included repeated losses, grief, divorces, redundancies, stolen identity. I'm not embarrassed to admit the chaos and trauma that I attracted to myself, I now understand it thanks to Dr J Demartini.

Instead of playing the victim role and blaming the other people in my life; sharing gratitude to them for allowing me the chance to live a more fulfilled life, allows me to take responsibility and own my power instead of giving it away to others.

Depression is simply nature's way of allowing you the opportunity to slow down and reflect on your life. It is NOT a disease, it is a feedback mechanism. It is an amazing gift, not available to everyone. The discoveries you will make and how you can connect and help others is one of the most rewarding ways to live a life

## To Date

From the days of wanting my life to end, to having no energy and feeling pathetic I can now say that last weekend I ran just over 9 Km as an early morning run.

I achieved my plan to write a book, and had the pleasure of going back to my psychologist and asking her to endorse it. She was joyful for my outcome.

My career is strong in large commercial organisations bringing successful change.

With hundreds of new connections and people I support, I have come a long way from feeling depressed in 2010. My work allows me flexibility and I love how my life is unfolding. I enjoy the moments as they happen, no longer looking for a future event to make me happy or depressing over passed events.

If you are depressed then I open my arms and say 'Welcome to the journey!' you are definitely reading the right book.

Thank you Hana for reaching out to help guide others. God bless you for your strength and resilience and for allowing me this opportunity to share how I worked with depression.

# ALOHANA'S STORY

Alohana Jackson
President and Owner, Healthy Living Choices, Entrepreneur helping others
find better health and create more wealth
www.healthy-living-choices.net

I didn't know I was different than most kids growing up. I would struggle with
being alone, making decisions and getting upset over matters that appeared
larger than they really were. My mother would give me a half valium to calm me
down and breathing into a paper bag would help get me under control.

My mother has been medicated for depression since I was born. Her mother
suffered from it as well. I certainly did inherit it by DNA. I remember my mother
staying in bed many days and I thought it was a migraine. Sometimes it may
have been but also the depression was a challenge for her to manage.
I did not recognize the panic attacks as a child like I do now. I just thought it was
hard to calm down after being upset about something and that was how every
child felt.

After college and living on my own, I did not recognize the debilitating effect on
my work until many years later. I never shared with anyone for over ten years
about a sexual assault I experienced at age 20 while living alone so that added to
my challenges of feeling safe and positive in life.

My first job after college almost ended in being fired because of the aftermath of
the assault. I kept it to myself except for the man I married who helped to end
the harassment and endless calls from the man who assaulted me.

My work history will show several jobs that I stayed at for a few years at a time. I
did lose a job at a law firm because I could not manage the expectations and did
not know how to communicate that to the attorney.

It was not until I was over 30 and working at another law firm that I realized I may
need medical help. My attorney was commenting on something I had done and I
felt he was yelling at me. Often it seemed that when I felt I was in the wrong it

was being shared with me in loud voices. Every time I was called into the employer's office my first thought was what I did wrong now.

When I told this attorney that our office would be better off if he did his job better I knew I was not in control of my emotions.
I went to the doctor who asked me to fill out a four page test. It confirmed I did and still do suffer from depression. He prescribed a drug, Serzone, which I used for three to four years.

Life became more balanced for me. But not before I was fired from this law firm for an indiscretion that I know was wrong. My work at the first was good and all job evaluations were glowing. However I was out of line when I sought out a part time employee to tell her she may be fired soon because I overheard this. Not only did I call her but I went so far as to track her down because I knew how to do that from paralegal skills.

It was the holidays and a relief to be out of the job that I was not happy in the first place. My husband was three hours away in another state so I applied for a job there and moved in 30 days to work as Executive Assistant to the President of an internationally owned company. It was a job I held for over eight years and managed better than any job ever held by me.

I stopped using the medication shortly after moving and found nutritional products to support my needs. I changed my diet gradually and began to exercise more.
When I divorced my husband I found the physical pains disappeared and I lost more weight. By this time I had lost 40 pounds and was close to my college weight.

During these eight years I did well with the American president but the Dutch president was a challenge emotionally. I was capable of doing a great job however I found he was a micro manager and wanted to control my work. He would not give me a raise one year thinking this would motivate me to be more devoted to him.

I was able to hide any depression and manage it far better during his tenure because my body was in better shape. I was learning how to recognize panic attacks and when I was feeling low. I would take action to avoid situations during those times so I could boost my own morale and moods.

Once I was invited to spend the night with a girlfriend and upon arrival found myself uncomfortable because she was choosing to have food that was not in my usual diet. I recognize that as excuse too to leave as soon as I arrived. While she was taking a phone call I was able to talk myself out of leaving and recognize my panic was unwarranted. I did eventually stay all night and had a good time.

About two years before I left my corporate job to become my own boss, making that decision gave me such a calm feeling that my relationship with the Dutch president became so much better.  To this day he will tell anyone he motivated me to change my attitude when it was my current husband encouraging me to go work for myself.  I did remarry and he has been very motivating and supportive.

Currently I am able to share my diagnosis and story with those that I meet in my business.  I have partnered with Shaklee Company to share their nutritional products because I found such good results for myself and my husband. I recognize the triggers that will cause me to be less likely to manage my emotions in public.  Being overtired, hungry, stressed or taking on too much work will cause possible emotional challenges.  I don't do well with confrontation and try to avoid it until I can respond in the best way possible.

My father's death four years ago brought me so much grief since I talked to him every day for the last few years of his life.  I let myself cry when needed and let grief hit me when it would happen.  I relied on good friends and my husband.  It is surprising to look back and see I was able to process the grief and continue with life as needed.  I talked about him often after his death and that helped a lot.  I was not afraid to share how I felt.

I find that when I am meeting with prospects and customers in my business that many have suffered from a bout of depression or it may run in their family.  Many professionals take prescription medications for panic attacks and other mental challenges.  Many of them don't want to take the drugs forever.  I share my story and that gives them hope for change. Since changing my diet, adding supplements (especially fish oil) and having a great spouse, I laugh more, enjoy life better and recognize when I need to help myself more.

One misconception about depression is that it is frowned upon to share that personal information with anyone. I have clinical depression and when I share this with other adults so many are so relieved to hear that they are no the only ones who struggle with panic attacks, struggling with lack of motivation and not able to control emotions.

I no longer use medication because I was suffering from the side effects of the drug. I now manage my depression with diet, exercise, supplementation and healthier environment. There needs to be more discussion of this topic in the public arena

## TRACY'S STORY

Tracy Wight CBT, RMT, ARC
Biofeedback, Repair skin, Build your body, loose weight, Remove stress
http://innerpeaceconcepts.com

My 10 year old and I went through a bad case of depression after my son passed; we had lost Mason my 11 year old and my son's big brother. It was a very difficult time of major loss for us. Carson began having anxiety depression to the point the school called me wanting the counselor to talk to him. Carson had refused to go to counseling claiming he didn't want to talk about Mason dying. He said he didn't want to be sad again.

It was hard watching him go through this so I put my emotions aside to take care of Carson. I had gone to an herbal school where we had learned how herbs can build the body. I decided for me and Carson after a few failed attempts myself from Dr's that I had to do this myself. I put Carson on the herbs I chose and began Biofeedback on him.

I worked on him daily if needed but always weekly. The biofeedback cleared emotional blocks from stress worked on meridians and acupuncture points that were blocked all these blocks were stress triggers for his body, all stress. I had become a Biofeedback tech back in 2006 because the boys were so sick with Asthma and I wanted to do things a more natural way. Mason Wight passed away June 4, 2013 in Colorado and Carson is now free of anxiety and depression and is doing well.

I still run him weekly to monthly to make sure the system is still building and he is still moving forward. I don't diagnose or claim to cure, this is just my experience and how I chose to handle my situation. From my experience I believe if we can remove the stress the body can begin to heal.

## RENEE'S STORY

Renee Seals
Trained Neuromuscular Therapist and Professional Health/Wellness Coach,
Holistic Health Educator, Detox Specialist
www.bodyrenewalbasics.com

I struggled with bouts of depression for several years. As a massage
therapist, I worked in low light for most of the day, everyday. During the winter
I would come out of my office in the evening after the sun had set. By
February, I would call my doctor, suicidal, crying hysterically. She would put
me on Prozac and I would take it until around May and then wean myself off
it. After two or three years of this, she diagnosed me with SAD.

I experienced some pretty awful side effects with Prozac and other
antidepressants like it. I determined that there had to be another way and
began to research other methods of relief. I began using specific essential oils
in my practice, especially during winter months; I also used light therapy with
some pretty good results. The books I read were extremely helpful. One of the
best was on using Amino Acid's to restore balance in your brain chemistry.

While reading this book, I found that I was a low Serotonin producer. Prozac
and drugs like it are helpful in the short term but actually will cause an even
greater deficiency later on because your body is fooled into thinking that you
have plenty of Serotonin and it does not need to produce more, so it makes
LESS. I believe that is the main reason drugs like Abilify were created.

The point here is that your brain does not have a shortage of Prozac. It has a
shortage of Serotonin and or Norepinephrine. Amino Acids are the fuel your
brain uses to create these neurotransmitters. Why not get straight to the heart
of the matter and take Amino Acids versus drugs?

I now take Sam'e whenever I feel the need for emotional support. In Europe, it
is used almost exclusively for depression and it requires a prescription. We
are fortunate here, that we can just pick some up at the store or order online. I

am a big believer in things that multitask so I like the fact that it is good for your joints and liver as well as your emotional balance.

I think that there are so many misconceptions around depression. Sometimes it's almost considered a character flaw when much of the time, it is a physical issue manifesting as an emotional issue.

Several physical factors were contributing to my problem, low thyroid function, hormonal imbalance and low neurotransmitter levels. Digging deep to the root of the cause, versus medicating the symptoms, I feel, saved my life. The only "drug" I take is Naturoid, a natural thyroid replacement that requires a prescription. Everything else has been addressed from a lifestyle change or a supplement.

**E.G.'S STORY**

E.G.Sebastian (CPC, CSL) Your Client-Attraction Mentor
International Speaker, Author, Client Attraction & Retention Specialist,
Certified Empowerment Coach
www.myClientAttractionAcademy.com

Back in '95 I made some "stellar" investments and lost all the money; left my
country, moved to the US and in a month or so I became so depressed that I
turned into a real-life zombie. Couldn't be awake and do things, nor was I able
to sleep. I'd spend my days in bed, trying to sleep... then trying to wake up
and forcing myself to walk or jog; only to collapse in exhaustion and
desperation, only after a few feet of jogging...

My brother used to tell me that it's all in my mind, and all I had to do was pull
myself together and decide that I can. Those types of comments were the
most hurtful, as I tried really hard to "pull myself together"... Prior to that I was
a business owner, generating $100,000s a year; constantly active; heavily into
sports, traveling all the time... I loved life; and even in that wiped-out mode, I
loved life (never had suicidal thoughts) - I wanted to stand up and live... but I
could not.

Went to several doctors, and each came back with the diagnosis: you are
depressed. And I'd get upset and say "I'm NOT depressed! I'm not suicidal, I
want to live... I want to do things...!" But all they wanted to do was give me
pills, which I refused to take...

What saved me? I met this girl, who only God knows what she saw in me... A
year after we dated I asked her to marry me (with the stipulation that we'd
have to sleep in separate rooms, as I'd die if she'd try to do something to me
every night -- I'm serious). Yet, once we got married, in about a month or two,
life came back into me. I turned back into a real human being. I'm an
evangelist for sex (and marriage), as it literally saved my life :)

Well, that's the beginning of my depression story. It's tragic, with a little
"funny" twist :) But, yes, I do feel like I owe my life to my wife, and did take

good care of her in the past 18 years. I never forgot how she saved me from the darkness of the depression pit. I wish I could say that the "blues" never returned - unfortunately, though, it does come back every year or so, for a few weeks only... and it's like cloudy days - I know that the sun is just beyond the clouds, and I just have to tough it out. I force myself to meditate, do yoga... stay out in nature as much as possible (take lots of naps in my backyard, staring at eagles flying, watch squirrels chasing each other, clouds forming and dissolving...); and in those weeks, unfortunately I'm very much unable to work - have to cancel appointments, and slack off with projects.

It's really debilitating. Doctors say it's some kind of chemical imbalance that happens for some unknown reason (maybe deep inside - ok, maybe not so deep - I miss my country, family, and friends - and this "baggage" builds up and knocks me out occasionally -- hmm... never thought of it that way - it just surfaced now as I was writing... maybe... I left my home-land when I was 23 - I'm 47 now. And unlike many other emigrants, I never wanted to leave my country; it just worked out this way for some twisted reasons...)

In my case, after 20 years of battling on-and-off this nasty thing (depression), it turned out that I have one of teh most severe types of sleep-apneas and it was getting worse and worse and I was heading towards a stroke pretty rapidly. This year around August I felt that life was leaving me - I even tried depression drugs... then quit after 3 days as they made me feel like a total zombie... and finally I listened to my doctor and did a sleep test (he's been telling me for years, that it could be the source of my exhaustion and "blue" mood). They found that my breathing slows down 1170 times, in average, every night - slows down so much that it wakes me up each time (1170 times/night) - and some of these "slow down" actually means that my breathing stops totally - 57 times per hour my breathing stops for 7 seconds or more -- those are some crazy numbers! No wonder that I was wiped out :(

It turns out that 1 in 5 people out there have some form of sleep apnea, but most don't know about it. It's possible that some people who are depressed and live in a constant sense of exhaustion, perhaps have all this as a result of a severe sleep apnea - it's a good idea to go through a sleep study to eleiminate that posibility. Now, ever since I sleep with my breething aparatus ( a CPAP machine), I feel like I got a new ticket to life - life is back into me - I'm strong - I can jog (haven't been able to do that in a few years) - I can spend time with my kids outdoors... I can do stuff with my wife that I've been barely able to do... Life is good. The price for all this? I have a life-sentence on sleeping with a stupid mask on my face, blowing strong air into my "face", ensuring that my breathign channels don't stop...

## J.L.'S STORY

Author J.L. Pitts
Freelance Writer at Textbroker
http://www.publishwithcfa.com/j.-l.-pitts.html

I have suffered from depression since age 5 I have been diagnosed with Major Depressive Disorder and Postpartum Depression I also have Dysthymic Disorder. I have been hospitalized many times for severe depressive episodes leading to suicidal thoughts, ideations, and attempts. I am living a wonderful life every since I had two ECT Procedures. I am on fewer medications and the ones I remain on are at much lower dosages. Still higher dosages for most people but quite a small dose to me.

I have Post Traumatic Stress Disorder also; it was the first diagnosis I ever had. I was successfully treated for the nightmares, flashbacks, hypervigilance,agoraphobia, and anxiety/panic disorder but was never relieved of depression, After 16 years of fertility problems and 3 miscarriages I had a high Risk Pregnancy but it was the happiest I have ever been in my life. I was diagnosed with Postpartum Depression at my 6 weeks check-up but refused medication because I would have had to quit breastfeeding.

I lasted nine months and my daughter started drinking from a cup so I finally was put on an antidepressant and that snowballed into Postpartum Psychosis. I wrote a book on my Treatment of Post Traumatic Stress Disorder It is "scar Wars Forged In Fright" release date January 3, 2015 and book two of my memoirs will be detailing the years I have been talking about the first book deals with my abusive childhood and the first 15 years of my marriage.

## CAROL'S STORY

Carol

My depression story starts with physical abuse at the hands of my mother and my brother, from as far back as I can remember. Beatings, threats, screaming, and put-downs sure do take their toll. I don't think I ever felt safe or loved, at least not by the one person in the whole world who should love you if anybody does—your mother. Where was my father in all this? With his head buried deep in the sand.

By my late teens and early twenties, I was having suicidal thoughts, which scared me. I told no one, but I did read up on depression and suicide. I figured since I wasn't making any plans to off myself, I was still reasonably safe. Eventually, the symptoms started piling up: long bouts of sobbing, sleeplessness, fantasies about suicide, withdrawal from friends. Thankfully, I did not turn to substance abuse.

Therapy helped a lot, but antidepressants did not. After only three days, I had a violent drug reaction and ended up in the hospital. I was OK the next day, but it scared me enough to put me off antidepressants forever. That said, I think medication can be extremely helpful for many depressives, but it depends on the cause of the depression.

I've known people who went on antidepressants to fix a presumed chemical imbalance and were eventually able to get off their medication (and not slip back into depression). The fact that some people have to stay on meds or their symptoms come back does suggest that the meds are merely suppressing their symptoms, but that might be the best result they can expect. Again, I think it depends on the underlying cause of the depression.

Because I wasn't able to handle antidepressants, I had to find other means to suppress the symptoms (no, I don't think I'll ever cure it). Several things have helped me at least as much as I expected medication to: getting a dog, strenuous exercise, spending time with friends and my daughters, challenging hobbies, various self-help books, and keeping my home reasonably clean.

I don't talk to very many people about my depression. Although I do think the topic is important enough to be discussed in the public arena, I also think there's still enough of a stigma attached to it that it could be professional suicide to talk about it openly. Yet if more people were more open about it, the stigma might eventually go away. Catch-22.

The stigma is fueled by common misconceptions about depression: (1) it's all in your head; there's nothing really wrong with you; (2) you can just snap out of it if you want to badly enough; (3) depressed people are low-functioning and unreliable. I don't know which is the biggest misconception. I've encountered all of those and others, and none of them inspire me with confidence that the stigma is going away any time soon.

## ANDREA'S STORY

Andrea

I recently suffered from short-term "situational" depression for a period of 3 months due to a business failure and loss of close to $80 000 (alot of money for me!).

You could probably call it an "Acute" case of Depression, rather than "Chronic" as it was very deep and debilitating but subsided once I started to get my life and finances moving in the right direction.

My relationship with my partner suffered, I was suicidal - a place where I never thought I would go prior to this happening to me (a psychologist called my personality type "Schizoid" which means I dealt with the situation not as well as some others may have). I always considered myself to be rational, and someone who dealt with stress well with strong coping mechanisms. I still do believe I am rational, but not so good at coping with a fear of losing everything.

My symptoms over that three months of depression were:- morning dry reaching (due to severe stress), loss of hair, loss of 10kg in weight (no appetite), insomnia, night sweats (from medication I suspect) only wanting to be asleep (sleep time was the only thing I looked forward to and I needed sleeping pills to achieve it) and basically not wanting to be on the planet, with a daunting feeling of never seeing an end to the turmoil, and the fear of losing everything.

One of my lowest times was when I attended a family function, but had to leave early as I could not find the strength or will to talk to people. I ended up in my mother's bed in the foetal position (reverting back to child) and just wanting my mother to be there beside me and keep talking - didn't matter what about.

I took anti-depressants as I was desperate to get rid of the black feeling I was experiencing, but I didn't feel they helped and asked the psychologist to change the type or dosage, which was refused. He used cognitive therapy and told me the answer was not with anti-depressants nor an overnight stay in Intensive Care (on valium or whatever they use), but a change in mind-set and to just deal with one hour at a time each day with small steps forward; to keep going and not to find solace in staying in bed - a bad and dangerous habit to get into. I knew what he was saying to be true, but when you are depressed it is like running a marathon with no end in sight.

I did seek help over the phone (ie beyond blue), and psychologists in person, some of whom helped, but some didn't - one psychologist made me feel slightly worse, as after 3 sessions, she ended up looking at me with nothing else to say - I think she thought that nothing she said would make my situation better. At that moment, I remembered thinking - well I really DO have a major problem on my hands.

Unfortunately, going through depression sometimes opens up another hurt and that is negative reactions from family.  Whilst I was lucky to get great support from friends and some family members, it does reveal sometimes, that other members of your closest family can seem unsupportive, as they don't understand and think that you can just snap out of it.  I was condemned for deciding against attending our normal Christmas lunch, as a couple of family members simply could not understand that I was still in "damage control" and could not handle stress (as with many families, Christmas can be a stressful time).

Some took it personally and as some kind of a cop-out with one member not speaking to me for almost a year which I found very difficult to deal with, as my expectation of family was to be supportive with my depression, and to understand that I was struggling. (I am usually the easy-going family member who goes along and agrees with everything, so they weren't use to me saying "No" and continuing to do so everytime they asked (expecting that I would change my mind). I needed to honour myself and my own needs and for once.

This is an area where I think continued education would be great ie. Information to surrounding family and friends.

I am pleased to say that I am "back to normal" and feel that I will never return to that horrible, dark place.  I learnt that my particular core fear is lack of security and support, and when that is pulled from under me, I suffer badly.

I think you will get alot of people responding with chronic depression experiences, but with short term depression and suicidal tendancies, it can be really scary and I can say that I have experienced that place of complete dispair and hopelessness, and lucky for me I got through it.

## ALDWYN'S STORY

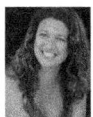

Aldwyn Altuney
'Media Queen' offering free publicity and online marketing training at Mass Media Mastery
www.aaxpose.com

I have had bouts of depression for as long as I can remember. I believe it is brought on whenever I feel overwhelmed, angry or helpless to change things about myself or the world.

Sadly, depression affects 121 million people worldwide and one in five Australians. It affects their work and personal life and can destroy their quality of life.

At its most severe, depression can lead to suicide and is responsible for 850,000 deaths worldwide every year, according to a report published in BioMed Central.

Depression can be a debilitating illness if not dealt with correctly. I believe one of the most common misconceptions about depression is that it is rare and will not happen to someone who is successful and seen as happy, outgoing and loving life.

I had a girlfriend who was the communications manager for a large company on the Gold Coast – she was outgoing, fun, bubbly, much-loved, secure with a house and boyfriend and loving family. She hung herself at age 31. Everyone was shocked by this yet it can happen to anyone when a deep, dark depression takes hold of you.

Depression can happen to anyone, regardless of sex, race or age. It is one of the most common mental health problems.
The World Health Organisation estimates that 10% of people may need help for depression at any time and as many as 20% of people carry the risk of developing depression during their lifetime.

Several popular antidepressant drugs such as Paxil, Prozac and Zoloft can have serious side effects such as suicidal thoughts or actions.
I don't believe medication helps depression at all – it is just a bandaid treatment and doesn't get to the cause of the problem. Most often, it turns people into zombies and takes the life out of them.

Personally, I have dealt with my depression gradually and gently. Whenever I feel like I've fallen into a dark hole and think that all my problems will end if I end my life, I pull my way out by thinking about things I appreciate, about my family, about those less fortunate and those I love.

I have done a lot of personal development work to remind myself that it is normal to have ups and downs in life and the more up you feel, your body will naturally attempt to balance your emotions and bring you down again. Depression has been brushed under the carpet for too long in society and not taken seriously as something that can and does lead to nearly one million deaths every year.

I believe it's time we brought the topic into the open and raised awareness and appreciation for it as a natural feeling that can happen to anyone at any time – regardless of age, race or sex.

Depression means 'feelings of severe despondency and dejection' and as life inevitably has highs and lows, ups and downs, it is bound to happen to all of us at some point.

The trick to controlling it is to recognise it when it comes on, appreciate it for what it is and stay on the rollercoaster for dear life. Because life is previous – we are all miracles of life and we will constantly attempt to strive for balance, peace and harmony. In that mission, there will be challenges and life will seem hard at times.

After all, isn't that what makes the world such an interesting place? The mix of dark and light, the yin yang of life, the waves we ride, the people we meet, the hardships we overcome.

Our struggles make us stronger and a caterpillar doesn't become a butterfly until it breaks its way out of the cocoon. Such is the path to transformation.

## ROBIN'S STORY

Robin

I suffer from depression. I do take medication and it has been a life saver. I do exercise and try to eat decent. I believe my depression has been made much worse because of early on set menopause. No one really knows the depth of my depression because I do hide it very well. I also go to therapy but feel it's not useful. My friends work just as good as a therapist.

Biggest misconception is..."just get over it, you can control it"

## ALEJANDRO'S STORY

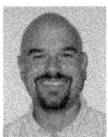

Dr. Alex Iñiguez, MD
SMILE International Consulting
www.smileic.com

At my 45 years I have suffered two episodes of major depression, with very different origins and conclusions.

My first experience with the depression was at the age of 22, when I was studying Medicine. It was about June, and I was immersed in the final examinations of the year. In those days I already was thinking that I had mistaken my vocation and that working as a doctor was not what I wanted for my future, but this is another long story that does not fit in this tale.

Though undoubtedly this feeling influenced that my mental status was not the ideal one. Anyway I was already under a tremendous psychological pressure due to the stress of the examinations. A few hours of dream, an inadequate and unbalanced nutrition, very little physical exercise and a lot of time seated on the study table, very poor social contact, and all that lengthened for several weeks,... until one day my mind collapsed.

I started having feelings of guilt, of uselessness, of failure, sadness, desire of weeping, negativity, pessimism, sleep disorders, chronic fatigue, etc. Until completing the list of symptoms associated with a major depression, except the thoughts of suicide. Lucky I never thought of committing suicide. But for the rest of the list, I experienced everything.

That situation lasted a few weeks, during which in spite of feeling really bad I continued trying to study and approve the examinations. In my ignorance, I believed that everything what was happening to myself was due to the stress, and that when the examinations were finishing everything would return to be like before.

I had time of thinking very much about my past, present and future life. I never commented on it with anybody up to one year later, when the following course I studied the subject of Psychiatry and on the topic of the major depression I realized with surprise that I had suffered all that process a few months before. It was a great shock to realize for what I had run through, and to have gone out from there without help. I was never asking for help because I was never aware, since it was never diagnosed. The problem appeared and disappeared. Until 20 years later when it appeared again, and this time much stronger.

My second episode of major depression was two years ago, when I was 43. Also it was in June: chance or not? I was in Barcelona in a business trip, it was a Saturday and I had to give a conference in front of 200 people. The previous night a friend phoned me to tell that the father of a great friend had died, and it was very difficult to sleep well. In the morning, while I was shaving for the conference I started weeping and trembling, so much that I was not able to continue shaving. I called my colleague, said to her that I should apologize but I could not come to the conference, and I returned to my house.

Four hours of train later, I took the car and went to the funeral of my friend's father. I was weeping all the way, but I knew in my heart that I was doing the right thing as person, and I was where I must be at that moment. The trigger end was the death of a very dear being, but I had been a couple of years under a very big psychological pressure: too many days out of home for business reasons, and a very high working exigency. I remember a February in which I slept 16 nights out of my house. The work-life equilibrium was clearly unbalanced.

In this case the diagnosis was very easy: first I auto-diagnosed myself; the same day a friend doctor agreed, just before the funeral; and during the following days my personal doctor, my psychologist and my psychiatrist (whom I knew because of this event) confirmed undoubtedly the diagnosis. I was suffering a major depression and needed a sick leave and the suitable treatment. Where psychologist and psychiatrist did not put so in agreement was in the treatment of the problem. The first one wanted just a purely psychological approach, trying to avoid the antidepressant drugs. Whereas the psychiatrist was pleading for the antidepressant medication plus psychological therapy.

Since I was patient but medical doctor as well, it made the situation even more entertaining. This way, during my visits to the psychologist I was always trying to understand his point of view with regard to the behavioral therapy and listening to his reasonings against the drugs. Even we were reading a book *"The Emperor's New Drugs"* (by Irving Kirsch) where the usefulness of the antidepressant medicaments is hardly criticized, with arguments based on the scientific evidence.

Nevertheless I also trusted my psychiatrist, and I was obeying her taking the prescribed antidepressants. In addition I also needed some other drugs to get to sleep and anxiolytics for the occasional panic crisis. Regardless the four chronic medicaments for my hypertension: I was a very polymedicated patient.
This second depression was much worse than the first one. Probably for the age, probably for the family circumstances, probably for everything or probably for everything opposite. The case is that it was well diagnosed from the beginning and I did not hesitate to ask for as much help as possible.

I honestly believe that the antidepressant medication did its function, but I have to admit that the adverse effects were important. In fact I had to change the drug in the middle of the treatment because the first one was provoking a few peaks of euphoria that were working against my recovery. The behavioral psychological therapy worked really well. Combining the face to face meetings with the reading of a book on the topic, I managed to change my negative habits into positive, and so making myself much stronger mentally.

Sport was a fundamental help in the process of recovery. As I use to say: "The best antidepressant drug is a good pair of running shoes."
Acupuncture helped me to better control the anxiety.
And the meditation together with the yoga were like an oasis in the middle of the desert. Lucky I have managed to support more or less all these positive habits, and now I go almost one year very well.

Another tool that helped me a lot was a simple App for the smartphone, with which every night I wrote a kind of diary of the things done during the day and, finally, evaluating myself with a punctuation from 0 to 20 depending on if that day I had completed a few items that I had established previously. For example: to have played sports, to have made someone happy, to have collaborated in domestic tasks, to have meditate, to have said "I love you" to my closer dear beings, etc.

And at the end of the month I can extract a graph where I can see the whole progress and the ups and downs that I have had. Because of it I can

affirm that I go almost one year very well: because during the last 11 months my monthly average has been between 15-18 on 20.
During this depression I was more than six months on sick leave until I could return to normal work.

The support of my family was not the one that I had liked, but I understand that it was very hard for them to understand well my problem because they had never suffered it. As far as I know, nobody in my family has suffered a depression. At least nobody has been diagnosed or treated. And, frankly, I am glad for all of them and wish to never happen this experience.
It was very hard for me and for them: I was feeling misunderstood and little supported, and they did not understand my apathy and my desire of doing nothing.

In spite of being a tremendously prevalent disease, unfortunately the depression continues being very unknown among the society and, for major misfortune, often it manages neither to be diagnosed nor treated.
I consider myself to be the lucky one, because I have overcome two very hard episodes and am still alive and being able to tell and to help other people.

Lamentably other depressive patients do not manage to overcome the situation, and it is very painful to think that probably with a major raising awareness on the part of the whole world, it is possible that many deaths by suicide had been avoided. Because of it I speak openly about my experiences and my learnings, for if hereby I can help other depressive patients to go out of the deep well.

Often I have wondered if the depression is, saving all the distances, as a "addiction". I mean that people say that the one who is alcoholic it is all his life, and I wonder if the depressive ones also are always in risk of returning to relapse if we go down the guard and are not always alert of supporting the positive habits and preventing the negatives from returning to our lives.

My psychologist, who has more experience than me, says that this is not like that, that does not have anything to see. But he does not convince me. At least in my case, I believe that if I stop being alert to my thoughts and habits, I have many possibilities of returning to relapse into another depression. That is why I continue training every day, body and mind, to be always prepared and in good shape. Since I wrote once: "I need to run faster than depression in order that it could not reach me in case it returns to visit me again."

# LINDA'S STORY

Linda Shaffer  MA, Ed S., LCAS
Licensed clinical addictions specialist.

My experience with depression has been a journey that I find difficult to track. I began abusing alcohol and cannabis in my early teens and still do not know if I was self medicating depression or just being a teenager. Addiction is depressing and I caused much of my own depression by abusing depressants such as cannabis and alcohol. I spent many nights high on different combinations of hallucinogens, alcohol, cannabis and cocaine until age 21 when I finally entered a rehab for substance abuse.

With 28 years of recovery under my belt, depression has not gone by the wayside. My depression seemed to worsen (especially after surviving a brain aneurism and subsequent brain surgery) throughout my 20's. By age 30 I found myself struggling to get out of bed, crying all the time, getting exhausted within an hour of waking up, irritability, and explosive anger. I was in therapy and finally agreed to try Prozac. It worked like a wonder drug!

I had energy, I could talk to people, I was cheerful and confident. I had no idea that I had been unable to process information like normal people while depressed. Suddenly, I was able to hear what others were saying to me without internalizing everything. I felt free! My boss thought I was a new person, I thought I was a new person.

Over the years, I designed my life in a way that would allow me to isolate when I felt depressed, set work schedules that allowed for naps or impromptu days off and avoidance of extended family. Now, at age 50, I continue to look for the right anti depressant. I find myself craving carbohydrates when depressive symptoms begin to creep in. I become irritable and short tempered.

One doctor seems to think I am bi-polar due to the hypomania I experience on some medications. This is a new diagnoses in the mix and I am not very receptive to it. The web of emotions is so intertwined. I am forced to look internally to honestly sort out my 50 year old female hormones, my addictive personality, and my depressive disorder. It is exhausting to stay on top of it, but the alternative is suicidal ideation, isolation or return to substance use. I am currently feeling pretty good and am on an anti-depressant. I also attend yoga, and practice mindfulness/meditation.

## CHRIS'S STORY

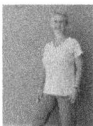

Chris Kirschbaum
Natural Health Educator
mydoterra.com/oilsedu


At this point in my life, I am grateful to share my journey with depression. It is simply that; "my" journey through depression, searching, learning and not giving up. These years of my life are the chapters which I would have preferred to skip, but as I rewind, I find that even though what others experience is different and unique to them, in many ways, we are the same. We are always seeking answers and learning from our experiences and pursuing balance in a healthy mind, body, and emotions.

This opportunity has allowed me to reflect and take inventory on the past 20 years of my life and it is empowering to share. Phrases of inspiration and moments of encouragement are what have propelled me to the next point of discovery. My insights and what follows are dedicated to my children and their children in effort to provide hope and induce resilience.

Living in Alaska for 26 years, I thought I had adapted to the long and dark winter season and as a busy mother of four children ranging from tots to teens, I found myself extremely sleep deprived. This particular winter I lost my mother to cancer and the depression began to envelop me. It was strongly apparent to me that my life goal became SLEEP, getting out of bed and avoiding the daily tasks of living became the largest of chores.

The once enjoyable early morning religion class that I taught now left me exhausted and emotional. At this point in my life I was unaware of any genetic correlation to my depression being that my mother was adopted. I had not access to family history nor had experienced any drastic symptoms in my life up until this point. However, at the age of 41 I began experiencing headaches with my menstrual cycle and definite mood swings, the kind that leave you irritated at the sound of someone's breathing.

In addition to my mood swings I didn't realize I was transitioning into early menopause. As you can imagine being a mother and having teens of my own, undertaking these these mood swings was something I could not emotionally afford. Although I did confide my feeling with my husband and close friends, I opted to keep my thoughts to myself. Just to give you a point of reference I remember my husband asked if he could join me in the doctor's office to which I declined. When finished I was sad and hurt that he didn't come in. It was apparent to me that I was emotional unstable. How mixed up is that?

Searching for relief from my downward spirals, as well as continuous exhaustion and lack of desire, I first went to my good friend who was taking anti-depressants. Telling her that covering up my symptoms didn't work any more and recognizing that I was truly desperate, she encouraged me to consult a doctor for relief. With her support and my husbands approval I was still very hesitant and afraid to try any drugs.

Recognizing the signs and tired of the emotional pain, I succumbed to the doctor who first prescribed Prozac. Not liking the results I was seeking, she then prescribed one other anti-depressant before we settled on Zoloft. It took about three weeks before I felt a difference. The main benefit I received was that I was not as emotional. I didn't have to spend three days in a mental distress. On the drug, when anyone would say something that might make me feel bad, my mind and emotions would respond, "they'll regret it" and accept that time would work itself out and not to worry.

Even though I was on Zoloft for about five years and felt that it was a welcome break from my emotions, I was determined not to stay on it fearful of the long term side-effects. Also unhappy with the current effects my search for alternative or natural solutions began. A natureopath doctor became a great support instructing me on how to wean myself gradually off Zoloft. Decreasing my medication came with side effects of dizziness.

I discovered the book, Depression Free Naturally, by Joan Mathews Larson PHD, in my doctor's office. Also Carol Tuttle's book, "Remembering Wholeness" and Marie Osmond's, "Behind the Smile, My Journey Out of Postpartum Depression" were helpful books. I researched articles on various methods such as tapping and meditation. This knowledge and research inspired me not to give up.

Mainly I concentrated on supplements such as Fish oil, L-Tyrosine, 5HTP, and vitamin D was part of the regimen. It helped me to be busy to feel productive if I could just get up and get my day going. It wasn't until afternoon and evening, I would start feeling better. Receiving enough light either naturally or through a full-spectrum light was important along with enough sleep and regular exercise. These health habits are the foundation to all good health.

In my search over the past fifteen years I realize that each person's health journey is particular to them and is their responsibility. The best part of my learning experience searching for natural alternatives is that the knowledge would come as I continued to seek. Whatever I tried I would usually experiment on my own for about three months on a particular alternative. I would receive inspired reminders of what I could try or incorporate. My yoga teacher enlightened me with the truth of her words such as "this is a world of opposition where you can at the same time seek contentment". This is a truth I had heard before and it propelled me forward to know that I was "normal" and needed to continue to seek answers while at the same time finding contentment in the journey.

At one point during this search for balance, there came a low point where my thoughts were very self-defeating. I decided to stop by my friends house whose mother, a foot-zoner, was visiting.   She then did some muscle testing on me and advised me to do a "Thought Prescription". She asked me to form "I am statements". These were the first I used:

I am honest. An honest person has integrity, is truthful, trusting, genuine and upright.
I am loving. I love myself and others. A loving person is kind, pleasant, sincere, and affectionate.
I am open. An open person is outward, just, accepting, willing, and listens.
I am thoughtful. A thoughtful person thinks of others, is helpful, responsive, sensitive, and sacrifices for something better.
I am patient. A patient person is peaceful, free, subdued, still, and willing to wait.
I am discerning. A discerning person ponders, prays, listens, is in tune, and looks for the truth.
I am happy. A happy person is confident, deserving, outward, light, and joyous.

I repeated them seven times each, three times a day, for 21 days. I had them memorized after some time so I would wake up staying them and also when I went to bed and at least one time out loud during the day. They literally washed my brain. They became my life line and truly changed my thinking to a positive pattern.

The second set I decided to venture out. Here they are:
I am grateful. A grateful person is agreeable, appreciative, comforted, praising, and satisfied.
I am healthy. A healthy person is clear, controlled, breathing, motion, and vigorous.
I am humorous. A humorous person is amusing, clever, funny, quick, and witty.
I am confident. A confident person is assertive, assured, confiding, interested, and wise.
I am ambitious. An ambitious person is desirous, eager, impelling, motivated, and positive.
I am tolerant. A tolerant person allows, forbears, endures, permits, and respects.
I am satisfied. A satisfied person is accepting, complete, content, empowered, and fulfilled.

In my continual search I just knew there had to be a better way. It was then that my daughter in law introduced me to LifeLongVitality vitamins with 9 essential oils, an EOMega and much more. I was really skeptical that these were really different from any other vitamin. Proceeding I kept on the regimen for about three months which to my surprise I actually felt more energy, less aches and pains and more emotional balance.

Regularly I had felt the need to take a nap but now I really didn't feel like I even needed a rest. I discovered that I was empowered and I really felt a major difference. I soon learned about other essential oils and how they affected my mood and energy. In particular I experienced and learned a technique called Aroma Touch which is an application of Essential Oils to the spine providing balance to the body creating a state of healing and well-being.

I use a blend called Balance in the morning for mind clarity and grounding, the Citrus Oils to drink and diffuse for uplifting at the start of the day, and my very favorite is Elevation, the joyful blend. What I have found that works for me, is only natural for me to share and empower others to experience the vitamins and elevating effects of the essential oils. This is my true find and the crowning jewel to my maintenance and taking the best care of myself that I possibly can.

The main element missing in society for people who suffer from depression I believe is STOPPING long enough to be in tune with yourself and taking the time and extensive effort to discover what works for you and never give up.

## DANNA'S STORY

Danna LaRue Bowman
Founder at Thyroid Nation
http://thyroidnation.com/

I was put on Zoloft almost 10 years ago. It did help; it does help to this day. HOWEVER, I believe it was a hormonal imbalance that went undiagnosed. As well as undiagnosed Hypothyroidism. I believe ALL psychiatrists and psychologists of the future will HAVE to test for vitamin and nutrient deficiencies, sex hormones, all thyroid testing, and complete blood panel. Truly.

I wouldn't have to be on as much Zoloft or maybe even none at all, if all of my levels were balanced. I am working on that, but it is a long process. It would have been better, had I been tested PRIOR to being put on medication. Many things could have been ruled out or diagnosed. My son has issues as well and was put on Zoloft 2 years ago. He is 13 now.

What started your depression if you know?
I believe I have had undiagnosed hypothyroidism my entire life and it is the underlying cause of my anxiety and depression.

What age were you?
35

Does it run in your family history?
Hypothyroidism and depression, along with some mental illness
What help did you ask for?
Therapy at first. I resisted medications for almost a year. It got so difficult as I was having a hard time with my son, who was only 3 and I was seeing and reliving parallels from my childhood. It was excruciating and disheartening all at the same time.

I finally decided to TRY Zoloft (and Focalin)  It helped so much in the beginning. Now, years later, it helps, but not to the same degree. I think that if I had had my thyroid and hormones tested, PRIOR to being put on medication, I would have discovered vitamin and mineral deficiencies and undiagnosed Hypo. I still may have needed a small dosage of the medication, but I don't believe so.

Especially with some lifestyle diet changes. I have food sensitivities and am currently being tested for them. Not to mention that we consume too much Gluten in our culture and that plays a big role in our digestion. We now know that the gut and brain are connected, as well.

I stopped the Focalin about 6 months later. I continue to take 200 mg of Zoloft and my 13 year old son is on 100 mg of Zoloft. He will be going to a Naturopath in 6 weeks and we will ween him off of it. It was MY idea to get his bloodwork. Not 1 psychologist or psychiatrist or therapist or doctor, EVER thought of it or mentioned it.

Did you get support from your family?
I didn't tell my family. Only my husband and close friend.


Did you speak openly about it or kept it to yourself?
To myself, in the beginning. Openly, now.

Were you able to 'cover up' the symptoms and work?
Mostly. But, looking back, all of the above could have been avoided and I might not have Hashimoto's Autoimmune Disease and Adrenal Fatigue now.


What advices helped you the most?
Blood tests. Do more than just the 'normal' TSH test. Run a full thyroid panel and vitamin and mineral deficiency testing.


What worked for you in the long run?
I'm still on my healing journey. Going gluten, dairy and soy free has helped. Supplementing with the things I am lacking. Trying to get those nutrients from foods, more than supplements is my next step.


What is missing in the society for people who suffer with depression?
Physical examination. Family history of illnesses. BLOOD WORK. Full thyroid panel. All vitamin and mineral deficiency testing. Neurotransmittor testing. MUST DO, before you take any anti-depressants or psychotropics.

## JEANNETTE'S STORY

Jeannette Mueller
Certified Holistic Health and Wellness Coach

Depression is something that I have lived with for over ten years. I had to learn certain coping skills to deal with stress and anxiety. I went to treatment and tried different antidepressants but nothing seemed to last long term. It wasn't until I discovered stoicism and emotional intelligence that I was able to begin really taking action and became responsible for my attitude towards life. Nutrition plays an extremely important role in dealing with depression and balancing out hormones.

Everyone is different and with all the science coming out about our unique genes, some of us are more likely to have a deficiency in certain hormones and neurotransmitters. Supplementation, and nutrient rich foods alone with meditation, yoga, and emotional intelligence have helped me on my journey to recovering from depression and it is now my goal to help as many people as possible be empowered to take control and escape years of suffering. I would love to hear more about your project regarding this book.

CHAPTER 3

## HEALTH CARE PROFESSIONALS ABOUT DEPRESSION

Dr Thomas Stone
Chief, Natural Health Advisory Board at Bajai Kalinga @ Las Vegas
www.drthomasestone.com


The root causes of depression, as with any physical or psychological imbalance may have multiple root causes. In seeking to help a person heal themselves, it is important to look at daily dietary habits, exercise habits, sleep patterns and quality of sleep, attitude and if they are violating the natural laws by doing medications that may be contributing to the new symptoms they are experiencing. Also as our staff psychologist discovered, many people respond to over exposure to electromagnetic radiations from wireless technologies in unhealthy manners. Just as the human physiology and chemistry is very complex, so it is with the mind and they are all interrelated and connected.

The biggest misconception regarding depression in my opinion is that it is still too frequently written off as a mental disorder.

In my opinion regarding the question as to the benefits of help that medications provide. The risks generally far exceed the potential benefits. This does not mean that perhaps millions of people have been helped, but in like manner millions have been harmed. Taking any medication to suppress or cover up any physical or mental dis-ease is prolonging the problems and consequently running the risk of creating more health issues than the original problem being medicated for. Medication does not cure depression no more than medication "cures" arthritis or the common cold.

Is depression an important topic to be discussed in the public arena? If we do not start making this serious topic matter more transparent we are never going to help people find their higher levels of peace so that they can "feel normal" and productive. Far too many US military veterans are committing suicide every day, bulling in elementary schools is so common place that public schools are war zones. Depression has no respect for age, gender, race or social status and can not be suppressed and white washed with current mentality of treatment and medications.

I am reluctant to give credence to the statement that "depression starts in your small intestine." Although we can be assured that there is a role the digestive system has, but no more than the kidneys, lungs, liver and skin as all body functions are interrelated and dependent on balance and harmony of all body systems to be functioning like a fine tuned Bentley engine in the Flying Spur.

There are far too many reasons for depression to list here, this is serious topic matter and definitely will have Hana busy writing more than just one book on the topic matter.

Back in 2000 when I was doing research for my book "Modern Foods...The Sabotage" there were 6.5 million people in the USA being treated for depression, and about 5% of those were children. I can only imagine that the numbers are much higher today.

The number one serious common link to depression or mania, or major depressive disorder (MDD) are intentional drug consumption of over the counter drugs (like cold, allergy and sleep aids) and prescribed drugs like antibiotics, birth control, corticosteroids, cyclosporine, Dopar, Lioresal, and ALL antidepressants including MAOI's (monoamine oxidase inhibitors), SSRI's such as Prozac, Lexapro and Paxil that are showing up in alarming increasing ppm's in our drinking water, and these serotonin/norephein reuptake inhibitors are dangerous in any small dosage. Also a leading drug contributor to depression and the horrible side effects is the popular stimulants used to treat ADD and ADHD like the Ritalin.

And here is a drug therapy that most doctors and the victims using the drug do not connect to depression and suicide, Synthroid. Yes, that drug given to millions of women for many years to treat thyroid issues, and Synthroid along with calcium-channel blockers are a recipe for serious weight gain and chronic depression, not to mention cancer and other ailments.

Alcohol consumption, even the alcohol in your favorite mouth wash, can trigger depressive thoughts and mood changes.

Unintentional contributing causes of depression are the drugs we get from non-organic factory farm raised GMO foods. For certain, if you are a non-organic consumer of chemical and drug sabotaged foods, like dairy, eggs, pork, chickens, turkeys, beef and farm raised fish you are getting loads of antibiotics, and potentially hundreds of others drugs and chemicals in your diet.

The most common drug in the food is a drug that has been banned in most developed countries, but is as common as the antibiotics in the USA factory farm industry. Ractopamine used to fatten the animals up for more profits is a proven leading cause of depression, heart disease and cancer. Yet people still line up to get their McDonalds, Taco Bell or other fast food toxic GMO food offerings.

Other causes for depression perhaps linked to the involuntary and voluntary drug and chemical exposure are perhaps just being human. Many young women experience depression post or pre-menopausal, some women experience levels of depression after giving birth, then again during the menopausal cycle, that is directly related to hormonal imbalance. And the same can be said for young pre-teens and teenagers and men reaching the middle of life cycle, hormonal changes cause mood swings.

We have been very successful coaching people and correcting many serious issues with depression and addictive behavior issues with diet, exercise, and quantum scalar energy therapies that work for the vast majority of people very quickly. Getting rid of all non-supportive and negative people is also something we strongly encourage people that are chronically depressed to employ in their new "happy life". We also encourage people to not buy into the over hyped MLM mentality of having solutions for what ever ails you in a pill, potion or lotion.

Chronic depression, or chronic anxiety are very important health issues here in the early 21st century that are too frequently ignored, or suppressed by the person suffering from the depression, mood swings or excess anxiety for fear of being pigeonholed as "nuts, crazy, different, dangerous" or some other negative label. The reality is that these imbalances of the mind are real, and if untreated, if not dealt with, can lead to real physical chronic diseases from obesity to cancers. And drugs are not the answer, at least not for any lengthy period.

Persons experiencing chronic depression, anxiety and radical mood swings should find a reputable Holistic minded therapist that has a solid history of helping people in a natural way rather than the drugs. It's incredible what exercise can do for a person with chronic depression of anxiety, a 30 minute walk works miracles for most. I also have observed that daily consumption of organic colostrum improves a persons mental attitude and creative thinking processes.

Mike Carey
Owner, Alternative Solutions 4 Health
http://www.alternativesolutions4health.com

Medication often creates the very thing that it is supposed to prevent, and the side affects are generally worse than the problem. As with any illness, it is vital to find and eliminate the cause, not merely treat the symptoms. There are many causes of depression, and yes, a chemical imbalance can be one of them, however, my testing usually reveals a poison that has settled on the brain.

Sometimes a deficiency in calcium can cause a problem with neurotransmitters resulting in depression. Many years go, I had two children with this problem and they were suicidal. Once their calcium was brought up to normal, the problem went away and they were happy.

I deal with people with depression all the time. Drugs, at best, only mask the symptoms, but often mimic the illness that they are designed to treat, and the side effects are usually horrible. There are many causes of depression, and many, many natural ways to deal with it.

One of the things that I often find is repressed emotions. These are emotions that are buried down deep and eventually manifest themselves as illness of one kind or another. I usually recommend flower remedies that will bring them to the surface so that the person can address them through prayer or talking about them and then letting them go.

Repressed emotions are also the main cause of Fibromyalgia, that is epidemic in the world. You might want to take a look at my website to get an idea about what I do. It is a gift and very unique. I have clients all over the world and I test them over the phone or via Skype.

Mary McKennan LMT
Specialized Massage Therapist
massagetime.org

Personally I do recognize that so many of us have accepted depression and so many other mood disorders as genetic flaws and have accepted it as "our life"...not our fault. We are so consumed with trying to manage our depression to get through our day to day lives that we are distracted from finding the root cause.

Often it is easiest and less time consuming to get on medications and constantly adjust or change them, rather than look inward (health, diet, exercise, attitude, personal responsibility) or outward (environmentally, job, relationship) on what we CAN change.

Besides, then we have our personal scapegoat and can blame the meds rather than ourselves when things are off track. It's generally cheaper to get on an anti depressant..then to overhaul your eating habits, join a gym, see a therapist, change a job, relationship or life style....another out for our personal responsibility, and plays nicely into the enabling society that we are continually fueling.

Kathy Cash RN, CHPD
Freelance Health/Wellness Writer and Consultant


One big area that is commonly overlooked is the occurrence of depression after major surgery or a serious illness. Interestingly, heart surgery patients are particularly prone to depression, which not surprisingly, hampers their recovery.


On the subject of depression after heart surgery. Both my father and my mother-in-law went through serious depressions after their respective heart surgeries. It was difficult on the families as well as the patients. In the case of my mother-in-law, she never fully recovered from its effects. If you talk to cardiac nurses, they'll tell you their stories are by no means unique. It's a serious postoperative complication, but the medical community doesn't pay much (if any) attention to it.

Surgeons, by their nature, are "technicians". They cut people open and fix a problem and monitor their physical responses through recovery. The mental aspect is basically ignored. Obviously, depression from major illnesses are more likely to be explored, but major surgeries in general… not so much.

Another issue I would hope to see in such a book would be the pros and cons of antidepressants. The general public is becoming rightfully concerned about the links between young adults/teens perpetrating horrible murders and being on (or withdrawing from) antidepressants. Are antidepressants being over prescribed to the detriment of the mental health of these people AND putting the pubic at risk?

<u>Jeffrey Briar</u>
Director, The Laughter Yoga Institute
<u>www.LYInstitute.org</u>

Depression can be circumstantial, but can also be purely physiological. (My father was a psychiatrist who passed away after 18 years of treatment-resistive depression despite the fact that he tried heroic measures - myriad medications, electroshock therapy - most without success.) Medication rarely cures but can moderate the symptoms - IF you're lucky.

More effective are lifestyle changes, such as: daily exposure to the morning sunshine (this worked for me personally), regular aerobic exercise and - perhaps most pleasant of all - deliberate practice of voluntary laughter with a group of other people (as in Laughter Yoga). Using the latter I have seen people free themselves of medications, as well as forming new circles of friends (Laughter Buddies) who create lives with a healthy amount of joy, where Depression became a distant memory.

Arnold Wiseman (MR PALEO)
Functional Nutritionist, Intuitive Energy Healer
www.misterpaleo.blogspot.com

If by depression you mean the "clinical" observation, and by meds you mean standard allopathic procedures, NO, they don't CURE anything, just mask the symptoms.... hormone balance, diet, particularly B-vitamins, sugar and saturated fat intake can all be CRITICAL...

When I was in my early twenties (we are going back a few years, lol), I was diagnosed as "Adult ADD". I am certain I was "ADD" most of my life up to that point, but anyways, I was put on every med used back then, trying to find the one that "balanced me out". After two long years of everything from methamphetamines to Ritalin, I said screw this shit, and started studying nutrition, for several reasons.

I am happy to report that I finally learned how important diet, food sensitivities, vitamin deficiencies, mineral imbalances, etc., were to overall health. As for "depression", "panic attacks", "fatigue", etc., ALL of my clients, with very few exceptions, start with diet, and my nickname says it all... I use adaptive PALEO/PRIMAL as the "base" of my healing protocol, which has nine progressive steps. I do not agree with those who throw an assortment of ideas at a patient, shotgun style. I DO agree with Hippocrates that good health begins, and ends, in the gut. We now know of the gut-brain/brain-gut connection. I build on that...

 What I have found is that "clinical depression" is often hormone, glandular (thyroid/adrenal), vitamin, digestive (leaky gut, as an example) and/or dietary in nature. Low magnesium is another common cause, including migraines, as is heavy metal toxicity. Classic "panic attacks" are nothing more than a hypoglycemic event, and are normally easily resolved by reducing the dietary carbohydrate load and increasing the saturated fat intake, and in emergency, a piece of hard candy.

I have also seen problems arising from the excessive consumption of soy, which I NEVER recommend unless fully fermented, and only then, occasionally. Women with hormone imbalances should avoid it all together. Drs. Hoffer, Saul & Foster, as well as Dr. Lee and many others, have made consistent gains in treating depression, et al., with nutrition.

Sherwood Grant
Owner of Simple And Good Enterprise, Wholistic Trainer of Health and
Fitness

In my world there are not so good days and good days, all the other labels
feeds the not so good days energies. When we can operate without believing
in such a word then we will have conquered first step to healing. Medication
never cures anything for that is not its design. I do believe we should have
more discussions about those not so good days that are still good but not so
good.

Chuck Bluestein
Writer of health articles and Independent TriVita Business Owner

Depression is important enough to be talked about in a public arena. Also medications just suppress the symptoms. In fact if you suppress something long enough, it can explode! This is why if you check you will find most of the mass murders at one time are by people on a medication suppressing depression. The biggest misconception is that depression is a bad thing. It can reveal physical problems (see below).

Psychology Today has an article saying that the increasing rates of depression are due to sunscreen (did you know that sunscreen is a drug). It causes you to get less vitamin D that is actually a neurosteroid hormone according to PubMed. Depression expert Dr. Steven Ilardi says the following: "Exercise is medicine." "We were never designed for the sedentary, indoor, socially isolated, fast-food-laden, sleep-deprived, frenzied pace of modern life."

He lists 6 factors to help depression like physical activity (exercise), omega-3 fatty acids, sunlight [source of vitamin D], healthy sleep, anti-ruminative activity and social connection. Anti-ruminative activity refers to things that keep your mind absorbed in something so that you do not think as much.

Please note that because of depression and a person not getting any medical treatment for it, it created a person that Oprah Winfrey practically worships-- Eckhart Tolle. Not only does he have best selling books but now many psychology articles refer to his teachings, like being in the present and mindfulness. Now he did not invent these things but before him they were not popular.

Karen Polvinale
Gentle Hatha Yoga Class at Body Language Yoga

I don't believe medication cures depression, I don't think it even masks the symptoms. It turns you into a zombie. At least that has been my experience with Big Pharma. I now use a supplement to help my depression and am so much better. So, I would like to see a lot about natural ways to deal with depression as opposed to Big Pharma. I'm very concerned about all the kids on these drugs.

I think depression is important and should be discussed in the public arena. People need to know that they aren't flawed if they're depressed, and they can learn to deal with it.

Thomas Hiatt,CWC,CPT,CNC,PT
Founder and CEO of Dr.Health Flex a Wellness Company
http://www.drhealthflex.com/

"As a man thinketh in His heart, so is he" , Out of the Good treasure of a man's heart so he speaks" I have often found that depression starts with thoughts and giving voice to those thoughts starts a cascading physiological effect. Neuro-chemicals associated with negative thoughts send Gut/brain messages. For those I counsel, I find it reverses depression when we "take those thoughts captive" and speak your blessings.

To change what is in your heart change what you say, do not act on negative depressing thoughts; filter your thoughts through a prism of hope even though your circumstances may not line up with your aspirations. I always remember that "I am not in control" of anything except how I react to circumstances.

These tenants are vital in overcoming the physiology of depression.

1. Recognize a negative or depressing thought for what it is.

2. Speak/ pray/ meditate on a good uplifting thought or memory

3. Forgive any one you think has wronged you (It changes you brain chemistry)

4. Exercise it lifts depression

5. Get 30- 45 minutes of sunlight each day ( outdoors) and supplement Vitamin D3 at least in the winter.

6. Laugh, tell jokes

7. There is a corollary between B-12 insufficiency and depression so have a uMMA test if you are not eating well.

Carol Leek
I help new coaches design their practice, find paying clients, and generate an income they can be proud of.
www.thisdayforwardcoaching.com

I definitely think that depression is an important enough topic to be discussed in the public arena. This is just one step towards debunking the stigma of depression.

I don't think medicine 'cures' depression but it can help in treating the symptoms.

I think the biggest misconception about depression, is that people who suffer, will "get over it". Depression also gets overlooked as a real disease and gets pooh-poohed and brushed aside as if it's just going to go away. We need more awareness about this disease, better understanding for those who deal with it, and for those who have it, to 'come out' and help others know that they are not alone.

No one should have to suffer in silence like they have for centuries. It's not a shame to have this disease and it is ok to talk about it. It is what it is just like any other disease and should be treated accordingly, in my opinion.

Patricia L McGuire MD
wholisticbeing.net

As a psychiatrist in practice for 30 years, I have many thoughts about depression.
Antidepressants are not the cure, but can certainly be part of the solution. Unfortunately, psychiatry has gotten so narrowly focused, we stop looking at the bigger picture--the one beyond the medication, and into empowering patients/clients to make the changes that need to be made in their lifestyle, attitudes, understanding, relationships, education and careers.

The problem that I see when someone is unwilling to try an antidepressant is that sometimes they are too depressed to take on lifestyle changes that would impact their state of health positively.

When I see someone initially, I always ask about diet and exercise, but it is usually something that doesn't get added/revised in the equation until a few weeks or months (sometimes, if at all) of feeling better. I support exploration and addition of supplements, yoga, tai chi, acupuncture, aerobic exercise, psychotherapy, essential oils, homeopathy--pretty much the whole spectrum of alternative treatments, according the belief systems, financial resources and motivation of the patient.

But, I will also say that at a certain level of depression, I definitely want to be able to rely on the medications that are most likely to be effective in a 6-8 week time frame. I have not found any alternative treatments that are as predictably reliable. I try to manage medications to minimize side effects, and maximize clinical efficacy. Once the depression in on its way to being healed, all of the alternative treatments become potential maintenance regimens.

Depression is a very complex topic. It remains controversial, and, unfortunately, stigmatized even at this late date.

I am a strong advocate for the mental health parity act, which mandates that psychiatric disorders should receive the same coverage from insurance that other medical conditions

CHAPTER 4

## RESOURCES

### About Depression

COMMON SYMPTOMPS

- Lack of motivation
- Lack of drive
- Lack of libido
- Lack of inspiration
- Constant tiredness
- Hopelessness
- Withdrawal from social interaction
- Suicidal thoughts
- Slow movement
- Slower speech
- May feel lifeless, empty, and apathetic
- Men in particular may even feel angry, aggressive, and restless
- Continuous low mood or sadness
- Having low self-esteem
- Feeling guilt-ridden
- Feeling irritable and intolerant of others
- Finding it difficult to make decisions
- Not getting any enjoyment out of life
- Feeling anxious or worried
- Thoughts of harming oneself
- Change in appetite (usually decreased)
- Disturbed sleep
- Neglecting hobbies and interests

## ANTIDEPRESSANTS

There are many different types of drugs used in the treatment of depression, including selective serotonin reuptake inhibitors (SSRIs), atypical antidepressants, tricyclic antidepressants (TCAs), and monoamine oxidase inhibitors (MAOIs).

Some Drugs Commonly Prescribed for Depression

- Prozac (fluoxetine)
- Abilify (aripiprazole)
- Brintellix (vortioxetine)
- Celexa (citalopram)
- Cymbalta (duloxetine)
- Effexor (venlafaxine)
- Elavil (amitriptyline)
- Fetzima (levomilnacipran)
- Lexapro (escitalopram)
- Seroquel (quetiapine)

SIDE EFFECTS

Side effects are common in all antidepressants, and for many people, these effects are serious enough to make them stop taking the medication.

Common Side-effects of Prescribed Drugs

- Nausea
- Insomnia
- Anxiety
- Restlessness
- Decreased sex drive
- Weight gain
- Tremors
- Sweating
- Sleepiness or fatigue
- Dry mouth
- Diarrhea
- Constipation

- Headaches

**Overcoming Depression**

Counseling

- Lifeline Australia
  Hotline: 13 11 14
  Website: lifeline.org.au
  24 Hour service

- BeyondBlue Australia
  Call us1300 22 4636
  Web chat 3pm to 12am
  Website: http://www.beyondblue.org.au/

Therapy

- Narrative Therapy
  http://encyclopedia.thefreedictionary.com/narrative+therapy

- NLP (NeuroLinguistic Programming)
  http://medical-dictionary.thefreedictionary.com/Neurolinguistic+Programming

- Hypnotherapy
  http://medical-dictionary.thefreedictionary.com/hypnotherapy

- CBT
  http://medical-dictionary.thefreedictionary.com/Cognitive-behavioral+therapy

Diet
- Balanced Diet
  http://www.webmd.com/depression/guide/diet-recovery#1

## Exercise
- Tai Chi
http://www.taoist.org.au/content/standard.asp?

- Yoga
http://yogainternational.com/topic/classes

- Swimming
http://www.swimclub.com.au/pool/index.htm

## Socializing
- Meetup
http://www.meetup.com/


## Other Useful Links

What is Depression?
http://www.nhs.uk/Conditions/Depression

Suicide Prevention Hotline
http://www.suicide.org/international-suicide-hotlines.html

Lifeline website on Preventing Suicide
https://www.lifeline.org.au/Get-Help/Facts---Information/Preventing-Suicide/Preventing-Suicide

Suicide Prevention
http://www.sane.org/projects/suicide-prevention

Author's article on Robin William's death
http://www.zujava.com/why-did-robin-williams-had-to-die

Author's article on Depression
http://ezinearticles.com/?Questions-and-Answers-Related-to-Depression&id=2728569

Successful People with Depression
http://www.huffingtonpost.com/2014/07/21/successful-people-with-de_n_5570970.html

## ABOUT THE AUTHOR

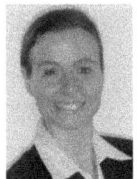

Hana Rubinstejnova was born in the Czech Republic, at the time that it was still called Czechoslovakia. When she was a very young child her family moved to the capital city, Prague, in search of better life opportunities. They moved several times during Hana's early school years. This contributed to Hana's resilience and ability to adapt quickly to changes.

In 1989, in her first year of College Hana participated in the events that precipitated the fall of the Communist Regime by the end of that year.

While still studying at the Business Academy in Prague Hana was determined to earn her own money and support herself financially. During college years she worked for Agricultural Newspapers, a Fashion Label Store and a famous local Chocolate Manufacturer, experiencing a variety of activities and working environments.

Initiative and ambition led Hana to take up a Sales Position in the Automotive Industry, and a Financial position in the Banking Industry, in her early twenties.

Predicting that English would become the global language of communication, she left for England and completed her Cambridge English Exams. In the meantime gaining overseas work experience in Child Care and later as an Office Manager in an Investment Company.

Inherent enthusiasm and ambition drove Hana to experience more and to grow, to study languages and to work both overseas and in her country of origin. Besides full time employment Hana participated in volunteering projects in Israel and in USA. Undeterred at leaving behind all the perks of a comfortable position in her own country, Hana's curiosity and determination brought her to Australia.

Overcoming the early humiliation of being seen as 'just another foreigner' Hana realised that Australia was the place for her to live.

With experience gained over a decade in many aspects of both private international businesses and in working for the British government, Hana finally decided to leave the corporate world and follow her intuition.

This guided her to study and gain certification in: Psychosomatic Therapy, Nutrition, a Diploma in Neuro Linguistic Programming, a Diploma in Life Coaching and attending various seminars over several years. During these studies Hana gained a broad and deep understanding of human behaviours, health conditions and ability in modalities relating to healing.

Always passionate about writing down her feelings and ideas, Hana has had articles published in Online Magazines. These attracted thousands of readers and have since been republished on many other websites.

With no true spiritual beliefs and an upbringing full of aversion to religions which taught about fear and money, Hana was an open book for spiritually sound work.

Experiences partially portrayed in this book provided her with further skills, a deeper understanding of life and refocused her attention.

Hana's contributions, inspiration, positive energy and outlook on life have always attracted followers. She has helped many people to regain their motivation to implement changes in their lives and so come closer to happiness.

As a Health and Relationship Coach, Hana helps individuals to rediscover their own life purpose, and the ability to heal and to live a happy, fulfilled life without the stress and burden of past conditioning.

Visit Hana's website at: www.HealthAndRelationshipCoaching.com